U. A. FANTHORPE (1929–2009)
at St Anne's College, Oxford, bef
Head of English at Cheltenham Ladies' College, and then 'became a middle-aged drop-out in order to write', publishing her first collection, *Side Effects*, in 1978. Her eight volumes of poetry were all published by Peterloo, and her first *Selected Poems* was published by Penguin in 1986. Enitharmon Press publish her *New & Collected Poems*, her *Christmas Poems* and *From Me to You*, love poems by Fanthorpe and R. V. Bailey. In 1994 U. A. Fanthorpe was the first woman to be nominated for the post of Professor of Poetry at Oxford. She was awarded the CBE in 2001 and the Queen's Gold Medal for Poetry in 2003.

R. V. BAILEY has published five poetry collections: *Course Work* (1997), *Marking Time* (Peterloo, 2004), *Credentials* (Oversteps, 2012), *From Me To You* (Peterloo / Enitharmon, 2007, written with her long-term partner U. A. Fanthorpe), and *The Losing Game* (Mariscat, 2010).

———

'U. A. Fanthorpe is an extraordinary poet, one of the best of our 20th and 21st centuries. So quietly that we didn't notice what was happening, her poetry changed the way we see, the way we write. Tender and funny, without show, without noise, using ordinary language, she lit with love the familiar world we had not valued enough, shook us awake with her undecorated language, made us laugh and broke our hearts in a few phrases. It crept up on us unaware – the transformation of what was possible in contemporary English poetry.'   GILLIAN CLARKE

U. A. Fanthorpe

Berowne's Book

Selected and introduced by
R. V. Bailey

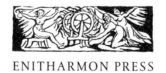

ENITHARMON PRESS

First published in 2015
by Enitharmon Press
10 Bury Place
London WC1A 2JL

www.enitharmon.co.uk

Distributed in the UK by
Central Books
99 Wallis Road
London E9 5LN

Distributed in the USA and Canada
by Independent Publishers Group
814 North Franklin Street
Chicago, IL 60610
USA
www.ipgbooks.com

ISBN: 978-1-910392-13-3

Enitharmon Press gratefully acknowledges the financial support of
Arts Council England, through Grants for the Arts.

Individuals contribute to sustain the Press through the
Enitharmon Friends Scheme. We are deeply grateful to all Friends,
particularly our Patrons: Colin Beer, Duncan Forbes, Sean O'Connor
and those who wished to remain anonymous.

British Library Cataloguing-in-Publication Data.
A catalogue record for this book is available
from the British Library.

Designed in Albertina by Libanus Press
and printed in England by
Short Run Press

CONTENTS

INTRODUCTION

U. A. Fanthorpe's seventh poetry collection, published in 2000, was called *Consequences*. Its title, the name of an old party game, suggests that nothing happens in isolation from the past or the future, a sentiment that was often subtly present in her work. It was certainly illustrated in her own career's trajectory. Her role as a poet began suddenly and unexpectedly, when she took a job as a clerk/receptionist at a small hospital near Bristol in 1974 – a job that would change her life.

But since, as she says, 'nothing happens in isolation', a number of interesting factors lay quietly behind this move. One such factor was the person she was. All her life, UA had wanted to be a writer. But she never thought of herself as a poet (she thought she 'wasn't good enough'), and she didn't want to write about herself. She didn't regard herself, or her experience of life, as sufficiently interesting to write about; she felt she needed more experience of other people. When, after university, a living had to be made, she became a teacher – a job that seemed to offer, unavoidably, a lot of people. But teaching can be an oddly seductive occupation, and it wasn't until sixteen years later that she realised all her time and creative energy were being used up in her work, and that if she didn't get out of teaching she'd never become a writer. So she fled.

At that time (the early 1970s) one salary was enough to support two people. The salary, such as it was, was to be mine, as a low form of life in the world of lecturing; she, the writer, would be supported by it, and free at last to write. It seemed a good idea. But inevitably the cost of living went up – and somehow a cat and dog had materialised, and they had to be supported too. And in fact the writer wasn't enjoying not having a proper job as much as she'd hoped; sitting at home over an empty page wasn't inspiring. Perhaps things would work out better if the writer had a job – but just a routine sort of job.

So she decided to become what was called a Temp. Her first job was at Hoovers Complaints Department; the next, at Butlers Chemicals, at Avonmouth. These temporary jobs gave her things (and people) to think (and write) about, and at last she did begin to write. She'd already written a couple of plays, as a teacher; now she wrote all sorts of things: reviews, criticism, even a crime novel. She wrote about other people. And she wrote in prose.

A second factor was the choice of hospital work. Each of her temporary employers had offered her permanent work, but she wasn't seduced. Then one day, sitting in a lay-by near Frenchay over a picnic lunch, we noticed an advertisement for a job in a nearby hospital, and this particularly appealed to her. Twenty years before, when she'd been at Oxford University, she'd been run over by an army lorry, which crushed one of her feet; this resulted in a three months' stay at the Radcliffe Hospital. She was young and fit, and survived the many operations, and eventually she even began quite to enjoy the prolonged convalescence. She forgot about her university studies; it was the other patients, and the staff and the system, that interested her. So, remembering the Radcliffe, she thought a hospital job would be congenial. She applied, was interviewed, got the job: as she put it herself, 'In 1974, having found that the way to get a job was to conceal my qualifications, I contrived to be taken on as a clerk/receptionist in a small hospital.'

But a neuro-psychiatric hospital provided very different experiences from those she'd had in Oxford. 'From my receptionist's glass dug-out I watched a world I hadn't imagined, of the epileptic, the depressed, the obsessive, the brain-damaged, the violent, the helpless . . .' She had never before encountered such harrowing situations; and she realised that if she hadn't, probably most other people hadn't either. And here yet another factor lay behind the scene: her father had been a barrister, and then a judge. From him she had learned the importance of the evidence of the witness. In the hospital, she saw herself as a witness, with a witness's responsibility. She believed she had to write about what she saw.

A final strand, that determined that what she wrote was no longer prose but poetry, was her interest in the way people spoke: 'I grew fond of the patients, who tended to come regularly. I knew about them from their notes, I heard their conversations while they were waiting, I answered their questions when I could, I met their relatives. Opposed to this talk, warm, lively, affectionate, local, humane (nothing brings out humanity like hospitals), was the clinical language of the doctors.' Which was, of course, prose. And suddenly it was clear that prose didn't fit: 'I was a witness' she wrote, 'and what I saw could not be described in prose.'

'Quite early on, after a month, I tipped over into poetry. I could think of no other way of responding to this babel of voices, this jumble of codes, everyone wanting something, and most of them held back, by illness or etiquette, from achieving the effective spark of communication. I was the translator in my job, and I tried to translate when I wrote.'

She always maintained that the poetry began at precisely 1.20 on Thursday 18 April, during her forty minutes' lunch-time break. She was allowed to take her cheese and apple and spend her lunch-time in a disused caravan in the hospital grounds. Here, surrounded by dead spiders and used hospital notes and lists, she wrote her earliest poems, in pencil, on the sun-browned backs of these hospital notes. That first poem, on 18 April, was 'For St Peter'. It was written out of a kind of exasperated fury at the situation of the patients. A doctor had been angry with a patient who had arrived five minutes late for an appointment: 'He had not seen that she had had to arrange for a baby-sitter and take her children to school and catch three buses in order to get to the hospital. His life was much easier. It's a poem which is partly humorous but filled with anger.'

It was just before this happened that she wrote *Berowne's Book*.

The poems

The early poems trip off the page. Rhyme and iambic pentameters were sometimes the patterns, though she was clear that rhyme wasn't appropriate: 'in my hands it was altogether too jaunty and confident for the circumstances'. But when the poems do rhyme, the rhymes aren't too predictable, and the thought easily moves towards a neat (and quite often surprising) end.

The 1974 poems are all of course apprentice poems, only the poems of a beginner. But this was an unusually assured beginner, for behind the poems lay a lifetime of commitment to words and writing. All the deep literary wells of her past life, 'great surges of Shakespeare', the accumulated echoes of etymology and idiom from Beowulf to Brecht – all of it washed over her in those early days, amid the strange dissonances of the hospital.

Not all the poems of 1974 were hospital poems. Of course the hospital and its patients and doctors provided a wealth of material, but there was more to life than the hospital. She wrote about friends, places, animals; cats and cows and birds, falconry and road-kill; about the Scottish midge and making jam and rehearsals of Wilde. She wrote poems addressed to the Holy Ghost, as well as to Coleridge and Sappho and Geoffrey de Vinsauf; she wrote poems from the point of view of an egg, or of birds at dawn. There was no stopping her.

Despite the high-minded commitment as a witness to the truth as she saw it, it was hard to be happy, surrounded as she was by so much misery. The job involved organising outpatient clinics, and as she watched the outpatients, she began more and more to admire their stoicism, their cheerfulness, their patience. She wanted to do something *for* them and, as the least qualified person in the hospital, all she could do was listen, suggest a visit to the canteen, show them where the lavatories were, and assure them that Dr X couldn't possibly keep them waiting much longer. It wasn't her own experience, but that somehow didn't matter. Writing was really all she could do for the patients: despite its self-mockery, 'The List' makes it clear that she wanted to do what she could to help, even if the only thing she could do was give the patients the dignity of a well-typed list.

There were advantages in her position, not least her solitary lunch-hour in the caravan, when she could work undisturbed on the poems that had been brewing all morning. All the much-loved volumes of the *OED* were available to her, in a bookshelf just upstairs. She had, too, the pleasure of an unexplored poetic vantage-point (in one poem she saw it as that of the flea) which offered plenty of opportunities for irony.

But she was lonely. She was the only clerk/receptionist, located in her own no-man's-land, apart from the nurses, the doctors and the patients. She described this herself:

'I am surrounded by people, but I'm far more lonely than if I were actually on my own. The kind of loneliness I experience here is a formal underlining of the fact that I don't fit…. In a way I value this experience, because I think it enables me to focus more clearly on the others. They hardly see me, because they are prepared to see me as an extension of the things I use: a telephone, a typewriter with legs, and an ear. I hardly see myself in relation to them, and therefore it seems easier to think about them objectively. So I don't try to fit. I don't really see how I could, and in any case it would be a sort of invalidating of my experience if I were to try. I seem to have acquired a camouflage without trying, and one which, oddly, doesn't involve disguising myself as something which I'm not.'

What she's describing was, in fact, what she'd come to recognise as the unavoidable situation of the poet; apart, even uncomfortably apart, from everyone else. She writes about this later, with feeling, in the case of the visiting writer-fellow (in 'In Residence').

So she sometimes wrote just to cheer herself up. *Berowne's Book* was the fruit of this impulse, and so was 'Only Here for the Bier', and a number of other witty trifles. 'A Letter from the Doctor' was another short prose piece from those early days: it's interestingly more acerbic than *Berowne*, and (unsurprisingly) focused on the words doctors use.

'The talisman which the patient must have to gain entrance into our Enchanted Castle is a letter from his GP. Without this, he won't get any further than me. Patients are oddly casual about this element in our ritual. *Oh, the letter?* they say. *Yes, I left it at home. I'll send it on to you, shall I?* – little realising that no consultant here will be able to bring himself to look at a patient without a GP's letter, to give him the proper perspective.

'The fact that these letters are often scanty in the extreme (*'dear Butch, would you mind casting your eye over this woman? She baffles me. Yours, Curly'*) is irrelevant.

'Sometimes it's the patient who has forgotten to bring the letter, sometimes the GP who has forgotten to write it. On such occasions I have to ring the surgery, and get a discursive account of the patient's relationships with wife, parents, children, GP, but nothing much in the way of hard medical facts. This, I always feel, will reflect poorly on me. Our consultant will think it's I, the lay idiot, who go in for all this human interest stuff, and can't spell a convulsion or a drug, whereas in fact it's the GP, a poor hand at dictating letters but avid for sympathy from a captive receptionist.

'Armed with this letter, then, the patient guilelessly approaches our portals. Vaguely he knows the letter is about him, but he has little idea of the figure he cuts in it. If he knew, he would give us a very wide berth.

'There is a special prose style which is cultivated by doctors. I have come to the conclusion that it is handed on from one generation to the next, and that doctors aren't sufficiently interested in literature, or sensitive to implications, to do anything to modify what they have inherited. The doctor himself, in these letters, comes across as an omniscient, sophisticated, Edwardian figure. He knows everything and has been everywhere; as a result, his patients seem to him rather pygmy figures, whom he sees benevolently through the past. He conveys this firstly through his use of nouns. To the doctor, the three obvious words you would think he might use (man, woman, patient) are all, for some esoteric reason, taboo. Instead he lives in a *Shropshire Lad* sort of world of *lads*, *lasses*, *girls* and *chaps*, with occasionally a backslapping *fellow*. Age has little to do with this terminology. At well over 40, and a grandparent, you may still qualify as a *lad* or a *lass* in your doctor's letters about you. For some time I puzzled over this phenomenon. Perhaps, I thought, it was confined to the very elderly GPs, who couldn't abandon the usages of their youth. Then I discovered that even the most recently qualified do it, too. And so the answer became clear to me. This is not a reflection of the doctor's age and experience, but of the patient's helplessness. In the doctor's eyes, the patient is an Arcadian innocent, probably wearing a smock and carrying a shepherd's crook as he rambles through the blossomy Shropshire meadows. The fact that he is a 32-year-old manager of a catering department, married, with four children, a car and a mortgage, doesn't disturb the tranquil picture at all.

'So much for nouns. But the doctor is a man of learning and doesn't stop there. He has verbs at his disposal, too. And the verbs he uses come from quite a different world, the world of Jaggers, the suspicious lawyer. Verbs are the cardinal points here, and four verbs in particular: *claim, admit, deny, confess.* Armed with these weapons, the GP need fear no irrational movement of sympathy for his patient. For the patient has become a defendant, and every statement he makes will be used in evidence. The unlucky patient, relaxed in the apparently sympathetic atmosphere of the surgery, has no idea of the deplorable role that he will play in the doctor's letter about him.'

Berowne's Book is UAF's last attempt to catch in prose the reliable absurdity of the way we all behave in our everyday human skins, both professionally and privately. That ironic glance would sharpen, in the economy of poetry, to something quite scalpel-like in its wit – and in its never-failing compassion.

RVB

Berowne's Book

Rosaline: You shall this twelvemonth term from day to day
    Visit the speechless sick, and still converse
    With groaning wretches; and your task shall be,
    With all the fierce endeavour of your wit
    To enforce the pained impotent to smile.

Berowne: To move wild laughter in the throat of death?
    It cannot be; it is impossible:
    Mirth cannot move a soul in agony.

William Shakespeare, *Love's Labour's Lost*

'All professions are conspiracies against the laity.'

George Bernard Shaw, *The Doctor's Dilemma*

THE RECEPTIONIST

The archetypal receptionist was Cerberus, the dog who guarded the precincts of Hell. This creature obviously cultivated the manner which receptionists are forced, by consultants, to employ. *No, you can't speak to Dr X* is the theme, and the reasons given will vary according to whim. *He's in conference / on holiday / seeing a patient / at another hospital / his car / wife has broken down*, etc. The one thing you must never say is that he is ill. This, naturally, disturbs the patient. It seems like a breach of professional etiquette.

Such Cerberus-growls are moderately easy to make on the telephone, but it's hard to perform them in the flesh, when the patient can probably hear the doctor's shouts of *No, I won't see the bloody woman. Tell her to come back next year.* Here the doctor, king of Hell, has usurped the Cerberus-function, and the receptionist has to modulate it into something more acceptable, like *I'm so sorry, but he is terribly busy until he goes away on his conference in Provence, but there may well be a cancellation. Have we your telephone number?* This generally works with middle-class patients, who have phone numbers, and understand what one is implying.

This is because the point about the doctor as Cerberus is that he Doesn't Mean It Really. Five minutes after the patient has left, perhaps in tears, he will emerge in a rumpled (Lovable Professor) state, saying *Where is she? Where is Mrs Z?*

Gone, says the receptionist, and to herself (*fooled again*).

Gone? I was just going to see her. Why did you let her go?

This neat ploy leaves one no alternative but to pursue Mrs Z. If she is middle class, she has already driven off, but that's all right, you can phone her. If she isn't, she's gone to catch a bus, to which you must chase her and then entreat her, like Malvolio, to a peace. Or, if she's a wily bird, and patients need to learn to be this, she is sitting in the canteen, over a quiet cuppa, waiting for the doctor to change his mind. You will notice how, in almost all these situations,

(a) the doctor wins, by being (eventually) magnanimous, by means of the lovable absent-minded genius pose;

(b) the patient wins, by forgiving the doctor;

(c) the receptionist loses, having become the scapegoat through whom the doctor apologises to the patient.

The receptionist does the verbal apologising. She also, by getting hot, sweaty and worried, provides a visual apology as well.

Naturally one tries to avoid this position by preventing doctors from ever seeing or speaking to patients except inside the consulting room. But this can't always be done.

The patient plays his or her part in the relationship, showing that the significance of the Cerberus myth is pretty generally understood. The original dog, you will remember, could be bribed by a sop, which was a wine-soaked piece of bread. Most patients translate this into the appointment card, which they thrust nervously at you as if otherwise you would bite them. Some of them see it as a magical talisman, a sort of Golden Bough, which they keep religiously wrapped in cellophane, in a special inner compartment of their wallet. Others, less tidy minded, have cards spotted with fish-and-chips, or with rings of beer-mugs clearly visible upon them. Nevertheless, they have their cards. If a patient loses his card, his behaviour becomes almost hysterical. He will ring up, and nearly break my eardrum with his wail of *I've lost my appointment card.*

Receptionist: Do you know when your appointment is?

Distraught patient: *Oh yes. July 11, 10.15. But I've lost my card…*

Receptionist: That doesn't matter. I'll give you a new one when you come.

Distraught patient: *Oh, could you?* (as if the supply were limited to one each, like an identity card).

A very few patients break away from this mystique. When I make their appointment, they write it down in their diary, usually with some such explanation as: *I'm less likely to forget it here.* And of course they're right. But how much strength of mind is needed to resist giving the traditional sop to Cerberus.

THE AMBULANCE MEN

The heroes of the hospital world are the ambulance men. Not that I'm certain that anyone sees them in this light except the ambulance men themselves. But that's enough. They always appear in pairs, stamping down our prim corridors as though they were wearing invisible thigh boots, and brushing off the snow they've dug through in the fierce July blizzards. *Hullo, love,* they say to the first female they see, utterly regardless of ranks and duties in this effete indoor world. *Hullo love, I've brought you Mrs Robinson.* This too has overtones of enormous difficulties overcome. Perhaps they had to kidnap Mrs Robinson, or drive through the night with her fighting off wolves? In hobbles the lady herself, and she turns out to be a crusty old experienced outpatient, who lives about a mile away in what strikes the lay mind as safe country. No matter. Mrs Robinson has been brought – and perhaps the traffic lights were against them.

Ambulance men probably have to take this line because of the real occupational hazard they must battle with. They are always late. Really, this is so natural that one should never mention the subject; in fact one shouldn't even consider it. But attitudes to time in hospital are strange forces, and ambulance men (and patients) are the victims. In sober fact, hospitals have no time. In my particular one, the clock in outpatients has two faces, one ten minutes slow, the other six minutes fast. This sets the tone exactly, but not everyone is astute enough to take the hint. After all, our appointment cards do mention a particular moment in the day, they reason. If we admitted that our sense of time in hospitals is anarchic, then patients would know where they were, and indulge in a sort of free-for-all queue. As things are, they're hopelessly muddled, but dare not criticise doctors or receptionists, whose good offices they are likely to need in the future. So they take it out on the ambulance men, absentee scapegoats. And even the ambulance men are only criticised behind their backs. When they eventually *do* turn up, it seems a trifle ungrateful to greet them with: *You've kept me waiting two hours!* After all, they are going to drive you home.

Women in uniform contrive to look either as if they're not wearing it at all, or as if they wish they weren't. Men have no such diffidence; they make the most of the costume, however absurd, carrying it off with an air. I learnt this when I worked for a chemical engineering firm. Men were always striding into the office in their full regalia wearing tin hats and boiler suits and carrying suggestive-looking lengths of chain. They were proud of being able to show off like this. The ambulance men are proud of their uniform too, but in a rough tough open-air manner. They leave bits of it off, or modify it to suggest their own individuality. Usually they appear capless, with sleeves rolled up and seven kinds of scissors poking from their trouser pockets. I'm fairly sure that they'd sport climbing boots and husky Aran socks, if it didn't interfere with the driving. When I first became a receptionist, I used to confuse the Fire Prevention Officer with the ambulance men, and greet him gaily with the standard phrase: *Hullo! Who have you brought us today?* This wasn't just a social blunder, it was a visual blunder as well. No ambulance man would wear his uniform as demurely, as conventionally, as the Fire Prevention Officer. It would conflict with the Scott-of-the-Antarctic image.

THE CONSULTANTS

The kings of the petty world of hospitals are the consultants, and by kings I don't mean modern democratic monarchs, but the authentically immortal sort, whose feet weren't allowed to touch the ground. I think, from study of their behaviour, that they genuinely feel that they have some divine power, which ebbs away if they approach too closely to the ordinary world. So they avoid normal contacts. The things they can't do are interesting.

They can't make a phone call. In particular, they can't understand the code system for long distance, but I suspect also that they're afraid they might damage their fingers if they put them into the dialling slots. And there is the danger, too, that they might have to speak to an operator, thus losing some of their virtue.

They can't write. This needs qualification. They can sign their names, and they can correct errors made by secretaries, but this is all. Certainly they can't write letters, and if they ever tried to make an appointment they scrawl something so illegible that even they can't read it afterwards.

They can't read. The only exception to this is the Monthly Index of Medical Specialities (MIMS), which they have to read so that they know what drugs to prescribe. Otherwise, the list of what they can't read is endless: GPs' letters (*What's the bloody man writing to me for? I can't read his bloody scrawl! You read it…*); names on files (*Where's James Smith? Where's bloody James Smith? Where's James bloody Smith?* etc.), when the file in question is clasped firmly in his hands. It later turned out that he thought it was the file of Geraldine Fitzgerald); and, of course, their own writing (*What's this bloody word? You can read my writing, can't you?*). Apart from this, consultants seem not to need to read, though I suppose that they study cheap offers and road signs, like the more ordinary human beings. I haven't yet come across one reading a non-medical book, and I have noticed that they are not too pleased by this sign of literacy in others. At one time I used to leave my current reading in an obvious place in my office, hoping to tempt someone to a comment. I varied the diet, as I hoped, skilfully: the latest book on Wilfred Owen; a paperback on battered wives; *Mistress Masham's Repose*; a handbook on English brasses; a biography of Vaughan Williams; the *Wotton-under-Edge Gazette*; the latest Dick Francis; but no one ever said anything. The nearest I ever got to a rise was when I put down a copy of *After Great Pain*, a book about Emily Dickinson, the American poet. One of our consultants happens to be an expert on Intractable Pain. He picked the book up, imagining no doubt that it was the latest contribution to his speciality, but dropped it with an expression of distaste and horror on discovering its true nature. The reason for this is interesting: as a sacred king of medicine he might have been polluted by contact with anything so profane as literature.

They can't talk. They are not consciously aware of this, but I have deduced it from the responses of their patients, who generally emerge from consultations looking thoroughly bewildered, ignorant as to whether they are to return, and if so when, what drugs they are to take, and what course of action will be taken about them. They tend either to ramble away in this confused state, and catch the wrong bus home, or else to ask me, as nearer the fountain-head of wisdom. So I have to bear the brunt of *But I told the bloody woman,* so that I can translate the consultant's esoteric communications into normal speech.

They can't listen. This, like the preceding, is natural in a sacred king. Secluded from birth among the high priests of his cult, how should he have mingled with the common tribe? Still, it makes for inconvenience when the common tribe have to explain facts of their trivial lives. Consultants have very little experience of state schools, social security, bus timetables, and the other immutable things that govern their patients. And the patients themselves are usually too tongue-tied with awe to be able to explain – or even to imagine someone *not* under the sway of these things.

Finally, like all sacred kings, their lives are ruled by ritual, and any contact which falls outside this area leaves them hopelessly at sea. They know, of course, how to talk to the various ranks of doctors, medical workers, patients, because the rules for such contacts are clearly prescribed. But how to deal with the patient met casually in the garden, who thereby ranks not as a patient but as a person? And how to deal with the receptionist when you stumble into her lair during her coffee break, when she generally considers herself to be herself, and not a receptionist? The most agonising occasions are the parties at Christmas or when someone leaves. Clearly the consultant here needs to show his flair for being one of *us*. But how can he do it? He gives the pathetic, stumbling performance you might expect from a sacred king who's just tumbled out of his palanquin and is having to walk on his own feet for the very first time. For the more everyday extra-curricular contacts, each consultant must develop his own pose. One of ours is so wracked by colour-blindness, hay-fever and other hideous diseases that he stumbles along, face in handkerchief, unless he has had time to think up some profound response (e.g., '*Morning*), which temporarily relieves the agony. The other isolates himself against lay contact by singing or humming. This removes the need, or even the desire, to communicate.

SRNs

SRNs [State Registered Nurses], like mystics, cultivate tranquillity. Obviously a large part of the post-Nightingale tradition consists of the maxim: Keep Calm. It's quite a familiar sight in our corridors to see an SRN peacefully meditating, while at her feet an epileptic froths and jerks along the floor. This is not as callous as you might think. There's nothing that can be done to help the epileptic while he convulses, and the SRN, as well as thinking transcendentally, has probably been noting a symptom or two. Fire Drill offers another opportunity for SRNs to show superiority to circumstance. While the rest of us are popping out of our doors and asking each other energetically what we must do, the SRNs are processing in a serene crocodile to sunny places on our lawn, where each will identify a spot suitable for meditation, drop anchor at it, and lie there becalmed until the all-clear. This beautiful poise persists all through the SRN's working shift.

Nun-like, she drifts above the turbulent intrigues of the inpatients, occasionally emerging from her rapt state to say *Now the best thing we can do is to think this over ve-ry qui-etly*. But at the moment when her shift ends, the nun is transformed into a maniac motor-cyclist. Leather-clad, helmeted, gauntleted, she streaks down the stairs and along the corridor, vaults aboard her moped, and is off to the passionate secret life from which she comes to work to relax.

This professional emphasis on calm leaves SRNs mildly perturbed by the activities of the rest of us. As I take the stairs four at a time in response to some urgent message, or sprint breathlessly along the corridor after a doctor, I'm aware that they are watching me, discreetly disapproving. Occasionally they will go so far as to murmur: *Never run except for a haemorrhage or a cardiac arrest*, but on the whole they see me as so invincibly other and different that it's hardly worthwhile their wasting good medical advice on me.

Our Matron, with a fine imaginative flair, has taken this concept of medical tranquillity a step further. Hers is directed at the inpatients, and her two cats are the operating device. Whenever an inpatient is likely to be particularly disruptive, Miss G. is discovered, in her office, combing a cat, or talking to it, or about to be placidly disturbed by its intestinal afflictions. *Come in, do,* she will say, *but don't upset Fred, will you, dear? He's not feeling quite himself today, are you, Fred?* (This is invariably true. Miss G's cats suffer from overfeeding, asthma, fur-balls and fights.) Greeted on this domestic note, it's quite odd to deliver oneself of raving hysteria. Most inpatients back away, and transfer their aggression to the Occupational Therapy staff, or each other.

The cats are also useful in that they afford employment. Quite a lot of time is spent in cooking for them (liver, or filleted fish); in carrying them upstairs to eat (they are getting too fat to manage steps easily); in opening and closing doors for them; in wiping up places where they've been sick. This is not, of course, time wasted. The cats serve to stress the safe nature of our world to outpatients, so they're good publicity. Where there is a cat (the implied argument runs) there's a home. Domesticity. Kindness, even.

I've never asked the inpatients how they feel about the cats, but I've noticed that they kick them when they can do it without being caught.

SENs

SENs [State Enrolled Nurses] are part of the magical world of our hospital, but they belong not to mythology but to nature. Like great sea-beasts, they have hearts which pump at a slower rate than ours, blood which follows a different rhythm. Their brains muse in the long submarine afternoons of their life, and no one from dry land can guess what strange thoughts are theirs. They stand immovable at intervals along the corridors, basking whales, arms crossed reposefully across their massive bosoms, chewing the cud of some underwater reflection. Naturally, communication with such creatures isn't easy. Our language is strange to them. Theirs has its own beauty, consisting mainly of variations on the consonants Z and R, which they dwell on with much force (and no doubt eloquence). If one wishes to communicate with an SEN, it is necessary to adapt oneself to the creature's own pace, and to use very simple words, remembering that they will have to be translated back into another tongue. It's helpful, naturally, to pause between words for this reason too. Normal speech alarms them, and they are apt to swim off at what for them is a fast rate, making anxious little motions with their fins.

These simple creatures respond, just as land animals do, to strong stimuli, and they seem above all to prefer olfactory ones. Thus flowers and infants break through their underwater stupor, and they will volunteer some comment in as near to our speech as they can contrive, such as *R luv–lee R–nay?* or *R iZ–nee luv–lee?* when a bouquet or a baby arrives on our premises. Occasionally some high-spirited youngster will run amok down corridors, whereupon the heavy lids will lift a little, and there may be a mutter of *Liv–lee, iZ–nee?* But it takes a good deal of energy to extract such a tribute from them.

In dealing with SENs, it's important to remember that they are, after all, aquatic, and that it is, therefore, natural that some process which seems simple to us, like walking upstairs or opening a door, will be lengthy for them because of the element they live in. Certainly, one has to exercise patience. But why not? We need to be patient with tortoises, too. And in the last analysis, SENs have nicer natures than tortoises. If they are able to understand that a patient is in need of comfort or sympathy, they will really do their best to supply it, with crooning inarticulate murmurs of *R–deeR, ZnotZbadZthaRt,* and other shows of tenderness. I should add that these creatures seem to be early developers, since they're seldom seen in an immature condition. We have one young specimen, which is a trifle friskier than the adults. At the moment it is even quick enough to move at the heels of strolling inpatients. But it's already clear that it is following along the same lines as its elders, and in a year or so will be as big as they are, another cetacean, basking statuesquely and ruminatively along our passages.

THE SOCIAL WORKER

We have only one social worker in our hospital, which makes me sad. For I feel, from observing her, that social workers can only operate in pairs. She's like a solitary crested grebe, indulging in elaborate imaginative rituals of display with never another crested grebe to encourage her with the right responses. And this makes her wary. She tittups along corridors, hoping, I think, to evade all contacts except what she would think of as 'structured' ones. She bobs into my office, but I'm no crested grebe, not even an inpatient, so with the shrill cry of *Morning!* she skims off before I can engage her in conversation. When someone actively pursues her for a talk, she refuses to countenance it in open country, where I suppose anyone might join in and anything happen. Instead she bolts for cover to the special corner of the lake (her office), where the proper rules of interaction may be observed. Watching her, like watching a crested grebe, makes one realise how little ordinary behaviour needs to be exaggerated to make it strange. For essentially she *is* doing ordinary things – talking to people with problems, writing letters about the problems, talking to other people about the problems. But each of these proceedings has been so hedged around with rules that it has become a stylised dance which, to the lay observer, seems quite remote from normal behaviour. She has a special voice for talking to patients with, for instance, understanding: infinitely tolerant, infinitely condescending. *These*, she seems to be saying, *are your problems, not mine. So let us deal with them in the way which I, after expert study of your situation, shall suggest.* The patients don't know this dance, of course. They must feel, as I should, like lumpish French peasants, suddenly introduced into a court festivity presided over by Louis XIV, and expected immediately to behave like nobles. But what can one do? The music says *Dance!* The tone says *I'm the expert. Trust me and obey.* So they do. And make a hash of the minuet.

OUTPATIENTS

Outpatients are either new or old. This elementary distinction accounts for the total difference between them. New outpatients are generally terrified. They don't know what we shall do to them, whether they will ever escape from our wallflowery portals or whether, if they do, their families will recognise them. This terror, of course, is natural. So is the way most new outpatients deal with it, which is to arrive in convoy, surrounded by sisters, uncles, babies, grandmothers – any relation they can coax into coming with them. Presumably the policy behind this is that if anything is to be done to them, at least the family will be there, watching the Jekyll-and-Hyde changes occur. The average new outpatient, then, arrives with a posse. So there is first the problem of sorting out which is the patient from among half a dozen possible candidates, all bobbing nervously about my glass window. All are sweating profusely, partly from terror, partly from the climb up to our hospital, which has clearly taken them by surprise. All of them need instantly to go to the toilet, and all of them are dreadfully inhibited about asking the way, so they have to elect a spokesman. As our lavatories are segregated, being aesthetically situated at opposite ends of the building, they get fearfully confused and even more embarrassed at being suspected, perhaps, of trans-sexual practices.

New patients generally have to spend a couple of hours with us. During this time they experience some natural urges: to smoke, to drink, to read, to find out what is wrong with them. All these urges they can satisfy, but only if they are incredibly persistent and brave. Smoking, for instance. Over the outpatients' doorway a Dantean sign exhorts: *You are asked not to smoke.* The daunting politeness of this deters nearly everyone. Keen smokers have been known to go outside in the garden in blizzards and thunderstorms, rather than call our bluff over this.

As for a drink: we have a canteen, so it's theoretically possible. But in fact the hours of opening are so cunningly arranged that the parched patient is almost invariably greeted with *Sorry, we're closed.* It's important to remember that our canteen is for the good of our inpatients, who run it. Their therapy consists of not robbing the till, boiling the kettle and selling each other a Kit-Kat. The needs of out-patients don't come into it at all.

And reading. We are generous with reading matter, in a rather clever way. You have probably noticed how magazines are fiercely sex-orientated: *Playboy* or *The Lady,* and so on. We play on one of these strings in turn. At the moment we are all *Autocar*; at other times we have nothing but *Woman's Realm.* This further embarrasses new outpatients, who tend to feel that we are probably not used to having patients of their own sex, and therefore that there is some-thing sexually *wrong* about them. The one constant provision in our reading matter is *Beano.* All our other magazines are the result of benefactions (which means that somebody has said *And you get rid of that pile on the floor, too*). But *Beano* is ordered and paid for out of hospital funds. It doesn't on the whole appeal to children, but adults will leap on it with cries of joy, exclaiming in polished accents *Ah, dear old Beano. Haven't read it since I was at school!* or else just sitting down seriously for a spot of hard reading.

As for finding out what's wrong with them … They are the raw material of an arcane profession. Our consultants may write to other consultants about them, or even, at a pinch, to the grass-roots man, the ordinary GP. But as for telling the patient the diagnosis! *Procul, o procul este, profani.* So the patient comes up here and stays for two hours, chained to *Popular Gardening,* deprived of tobacco, food, drink and rational company. When he's dismissed he's told to go back and see his own doctor (who sent him here in the first place), to find out what's the matter with him. Professional discretion can hardly go further.

New patients come to our hospital because they don't know what's the matter with them. This ignorance makes them nervously suggestible. They glance furtively around our reception area, drawing the most alarming conclusions. Inevitably, like any hospital, we tend to have some human waifs drifting around: a handcuffed prisoner with his warder, a defective child from the mental hospital next door gurgling unintelligibly to her nurse, a battered epileptic or two with mum, enjoying a day off from the Training Centre. And you can see the new patient's reaction of terror. *This is what I'm in for,* he thinks. *These are the people I belong with. In a few years' – a few weeks' – time I'll be like that.* The rather normal appearance of our hospital, its domestic cats, carpeted corridor, trailing plants and hessian wallpaper, somehow add to his fear. But the next time he comes (and it is of the nature of neurological hospitals that people keep on coming back), he has lost his fear, and his behaviour suggests that he is reacting against the feelings that he had on his first visit. For older patients come up on the spree. Like the crowd at Brighton on Bank Holidays, they come properly equipped. They bring their knitting, packed lunches, their own reading matter, and snaps of their holiday last year to show the doctor. They know the ropes, and impart a quite distinct atmosphere of festivity to the whole occasion. I should never be surprised to see a false nose or a bottle of champagne. This, after all, is a day out. Many of them combine their visits with a shopping expedition in the city. At the very least, it's time off work, spent in congenial company. For frequently old outpatients know each other, in fact the really astute ones wangle their appointment dates to coincide with friends, so that a good conversation may develop, in which nurses and present inpatients are involved. Alternatively, new bosom friendships have been known to begin in reception, especially between the mothers of epileptics, who sit placidly crocheting and comparing notes about the timing of their children's fits. Such old patients and their families are never at a loss. They know the names of the cats, and can fit their visits adroitly into canteen hours. They slot me instantly into the picture: *You weren't here last time. Where is the other lady, Mrs Robinson? Out the back now, is she? And how do you like it here?* As quick and expert as the Queen Mother at a garden party.

And of course, they all remember the hospital when it was quite different, and insist on describing it to me. I must have endured this conversation about five hundred times, but have still found no means of short-circuiting it:

Old patient: *My word, this place is changed!*

Me (wearily): *Yes, so they tell me.*

Old patient (not taking hint): *My word, yes. Now, let me see. The door used to be here, and the benches ran along this wall. It was all painted dark brown . . .*

Me: *No. Dark yellow* (not that I ever saw it, but I've heard enough).

Old patient (regardless): *Dark yellow, yes, that's right. And you – at least, not you, but the other lady, sat there –*

This conversation can go on indefinitely. There is another, cognate one, but with ecological rather than William Morris overtones, which begins similarly, viz.:

Old patient: *My word, this place has changed.*

Me (wearily): *Yes, so they tell me.*

Old patient (not taking hint): *My word, yes. Used to be a little country lane, it did, with bushes all along the roadside –*

Me: (faint with boredom): *Blackberries –*

Old patient (regardless): *Blackberries, yes, that's right. We used to pick them. Mother brought basins, and we'd make jam after we'd been here. And now there's a motorway –*

This remembrance of things past happens so regularly that it must be giving vivid pleasure to the remembrancer. But to be at the receiving end of identical reminiscences which one doesn't share, day after day, is an interestingly refined sort of boredom. Children, I suspect, experience it all the time, but adults, sadly, know only how to inflict it.

For such experienced patients time doesn't matter. Occasionally, misled by experiences with new patients, I attempt to apologise for their having to wait so long. But this interpretation is kindly brushed aside: *Don't give it a thought, dear. I can wait all day here. So nice and comfortable as it now is, mind. Not like when –* and off they go again. New patients point to the rather startling inconsistencies of our reception clock, or to the one on the distant horizon, which has stopped entirely and has a large hole where two o'clock ought to be. Old patients regard this with complete equanimity, as they do their health. For, although they come to us regularly because of the illness, they're not in anyway perturbed by it. Most of them know far more about it than their doctors; like Mrs Bennett's nerves, it has been their friend for many years. They have learnt to live with it, and have ceased to expect that any revolutionary new treatment is going to make much difference. I quite often get the impression that far from coming to the hospital for help, there are really coming to reassure the doctor. *Look,* they say, in effect, *this isn't too bad. I can live with it. Don't you worry too much about people like us. We're all right.*

INPATIENTS

Our inpatients are the experienced sort, and therefore, like seasoned prisoners, know how to make themselves comfortable. They have either an intractable but not incapacitating illness of some sort, on which they can speak to the doctor with a modest lay authority, or else some unmanageable cast of mind which has tempted psychiatrists to try many different types of treatment on them; but unsuccessfully, of course, or they wouldn't have come to us. As a result they are all, in medical language, interesting cases. They are, generally, moderately fit; walking wounded, quite often, even, running wounded. And they are mostly aged between 18 and 50. Younger than 18 would mean that they were altogether too vulnerable. Life in our hospital can sometimes resemble an XX film, and you have to be reasonably well over the age of consent before being allowed near it. As for the over-50s: I doubt whether many of them would be able to sustain the sort of strenuous hi-jinks which is the inpatient way of life.

On the whole, then, they are moderately healthy; there is a certain variety of sex and age; they have, in fact though not officially, nothing at all to do, and they stay with us for a long time, a year and upwards. The analogy is obvious. These are like guests at some aristocratic houseparty in Huxley, or the idle rich at a luxurious spa in pre-war Germany. The realisation takes some of them by surprise. Having been deposited by loving relations amidst floods of tears and confusion about where to leave the suitcases, they expect something frightful to happen to them, and are baffled by the unstructured life, the absence of notices, injections, white-coated technicians; the place doesn't even *smell* like a hospital. They will make a habit of passing by my office on their first day and asking me if they may do something quite normal, like making a phone-call or posting a letter. My utter ignorance of any rules (inpatients are no part of my official work) disturbs them further. *This place*, they obviously feel, *ought to be like a school. Somebody ought to tell me what to do. I may be disobeying a rule.* Such is the state of mind in which they arrive.

In a few days, however, they will have adapted to the life: *Keep Fit with Eileen Fowler* in the women's ward; badminton, croquet, or a mild form of cricket if it's fine, and snooker, ping-pong, or TV if it's wet. There are other amusements, called occupational therapy: these are chiefly cooking for the ladies, which is done in a matey, WI way, with plenty of companionship and laughter about buns-in-the-oven; and gardening for the gentlemen (this means smoking among the tomato plants in the tiny greenhouse). These occupations look like work, and are, of course, related to the hard slog one does in one's own home. But it's obvious that, in this jolly company, they are a great deal more fun. It is, in fact, a good way of getting rid of the patients for major chunks of the day, as patients actually in the hospital tend to be a nuisance, asking for pills, having fits, breaking windows, and just passing the time. In the canteen, however, they are responsible for money, and this is felt to be good for them. I seldom visit the canteen (I can't afford its inflated prices), but when I do I'm interested by the absence of any feeling of economic pressure. Much of the time is spent waiting for the kettle to boil (they obviously have a special slow-boiling sort), or washing up in a slow-motion manner, with thoughts elsewhere. Outpatients wanting a quick cuppa between having an EEG and seeing the doctor nearly always find that by the time the cup is washed, kettle boiled, tea made and poured out, some harassed person (me) has to come over to fish them out for the next act in the drama.

I should like to be able to spend more time with the inpatients. Our contacts, once they've established themselves, are confined to *Good morning* and *Have I seen Charles?* and *Will I post this?* In the world of the hospital, the receptionist has it brought forcibly home to her that she is merely Rosencrantz and Guildenstern,

> '. . . an attendant lord, one that will do
> To swell progress, start a scene or two'.

For the emotional life of the inpatients, which is the real dynamic of the whole place, doesn't start until she has left the building. But from five in the afternoon to nine in the morning, and all day as well at weekends, the inpatients' emotional kettle is perpetually on the boil. When I get back, I find that they have taken overdoses (in hospital parlance one doesn't *attempt suicide*, one *takes an overdose* – a subtle but important distinction), run away, smuggled gin into the canteen, set fire to themselves, broken the greenhouse windows, trodden on the cat, been rude to Matron, been found Alone Together in the television hut … You get the flavour of the enterprise? In general, they can commit all the sins available to girls at a good boarding school, but with the extra awfulness of the adult, married, and, in some indefinable way, ill. So when the receptionist clocks in at nine, hopeful of at least some mild escapade to relieve the tedium of Monday morning, everyone has suffered so intensely that no one wants to talk of it. The nurses shut themselves into Matron's office and gossip about it endlessly (this is called *making the report*); and the patients crawl about with emotional hangovers, sulky, lethargic, and trying to get out of their turn to run the canteen. For the receptionist it's like meeting all the characters in a play during the interval, and not finding out the plot until three months later.

So far I have written as if the patients aren't ill, and in some ways it's hard to remember that they are. Not many of them display the visible signs of distress – the bandage, crutch, dark glasses – that automatically make it a little easier for us to be considerate. But they are ill; that's why they are in hospital. Sometimes the weather stresses this more clearly than anything. Most of us tend to feel reasonably cheerful in sunny weather, and to take a turn towards melancholy when rain sets in. Our depressive patients underline this natural tendency. On rainy days they can't bear themselves. If there are few outpatients, they will come into the reception area, as a nurse-free zone, where no one will bother them, and cry quietly and hopelessly. Noisier patients will batter on the nurses' office door, demanding stronger and different pills. Male patients quarrel with each other venomously, and then seek comfort and reassurance from the women doctors. It's all reminiscent of Chekhov, except that Chekhov doesn't on the whole include a corps of ordinary technicians and typists who are trying to slog on with their everyday work, distinguishing *alpha* from *theta*, changing a typewriter ribbon, while the emotional thunderstorm reigns.

The drama of the inpatients' life contains another essential element: their relations. These people – parents, spouses, children, friends and lovers – don't confine themselves to compassionate noises off, as perhaps the relations of more orthodox patients do. These ones are infected by the hectic passions that flicker inside our walls, and respond in kind. They bombard the place with huge, expensive bouquets and telegrams, they take overdoses at home, they dispose of their children or the business, run off with the lover, burst into tears all over the consultants. And they do these things with a gusto that suggests that they enjoy doing them, that they never did them before.

At first I was baffled by all this. Why did the inpatients and their families live such passionate lives? Was it that, perhaps, everyone carried on like this, all over England and Wales, and I never noticed it before? Finally the acceptable answer dawned on me, when I realised that all the time I was thinking in terms of Shakespeare or Chekhov. What, after all, is the essential element in acting? It is, of course, the audience. You can have a play without actors, I suspect, but an audience *creates* a play. I've often seen this done by, for instance, a crowd waiting for a procession to pass. So here we have an audience of a particularly skilled and sympathetic kind: doctors and nurses, and inpatients with all the time in the world for the analysis of emotion. The play's structure is really more reminiscent of Racine than of any other dramatist. After an emotional crisis the participants go their separate ways, one for a conference with Dr X, the other for a session with Sister Y. They discuss the event in detail with these confidantes: *Why did I behave in this way? What did he mean by that word? What shades of meaning may be attached to his action when he… ?* And so on. It's a perfect activity for the leisured classes.

Like other forms of medical treatment, living in our hospital is addiction-forming. A really experienced inpatient has been with us so long, and adjusted so well to our emotional climate, that he ceases to regard the world outside seriously as a place where one could live. Then comes the awful day. To me, watching from the sidelines, it always has overtones of those tragic scenes at the dissolution of the monasteries, when members of religious orders who had never lived as adults in the lay world, and had never wanted to, were suddenly forced into it. The doctors have decided that they can't do any more for Charles; or alternatively, they can, but there is another patient waiting to come in who needs the accommodation more urgently (this generally means that he is the relation of the doctor, or the patient of a close consultant friend). So Charles is told that he is cured. However this is put, it comes as a fearful shock to a patient who has stayed for any length of time in a hospital, and he tries to defer it by all sorts of stratagems: wife on holiday, transport difficulties, cold developing, and so on. When finally he goes, he will slip away sadly and unobtrusively. A rare and beautiful experience is over, which no one in the outside world will ever understand.

Old inpatients revisit us. The formal reason given is for check-ups, but it's quite plain that they return, like old boys to their school, to see how far it's deteriorated since their day. They will test the atmosphere in the canteen, swap smutty jokes with the present inmates about the nurses' sex lives, address the cats effusively (though previously on mere kicking terms with them), get a handshake or a kiss from the doctors, and catch up with me, telling me that the present inmates aren't a patch on the racy lot they had in 1967.

And yet, and yet, these people suffer. They have strange compulsions of the mind, which make them desperately, unbearably sad; or which reduce them to the point where every object in their homes, every part of their body, is hedged about by rituals so elaborate and essential that it may take them hours to get dressed. These patients endure forces of the imagination which it's almost impossible for the modern mind to begin to grasp. The ancients could, I think. By saying that a man was in the grip of the Eumenides or the Erinyes or demons or witches, you left scope for the unbelievably awful to happen to people. We can't do that. We have to believe that it's the product of his early training, or that it's part of his gene inheritance from his family. More optimistic than our ancestors, we prefer the formula: if it's there in his mind, something put it there. And if something put it there, we can take it out. So our doctors try, by a combination of surgery and psychotherapy. Sometimes it works, at least in the rarefied atmosphere of our hospital. And if it doesn't work at home – well, you can't have everything, can you? My un-medical mind finds an illicit pleasure in the case histories of the obsessive, like the sort of pleasure you get from contemplating a beautiful poisonous toadstool, or a beautiful poisonous snake. These histories *are* beautiful. They have a special logic, of a kind that primitive societies would recognise. They are about serious taboos – not committing incest, not killing one's mother, not breaking the code of purity. But instead of belonging to the world of primitive societies, they belong to the world of supermarkets, clean-your-car-on-a-Sunday-morning, fish-and-chips-with-vinegar, social security and social snoopers, dustbins and babies and electric cookers, that most of us inhabit. And the elaborate structures of their rituals rise, barbaric as the sacrificial step-pyramids of the Aztecs, out of suburban sitting-rooms.

Poems

A GARDENER

Ours are a job lot
From the Funny Farm: shambling gangs
Of overgrown dwarfs, waiting
To be told what to do,

Or austere, executive Scotsmen,
Who issue crisp, instantly misunderstood orders,
Decamping before incomprehension
Becomes too obvious.

This one materialised
Pruning an abandoned rambler
With placid accuracy.

We spoke. I asked, he taught me
To know growths of different years,
How each year sets its signature on roses
Like hallmarked silver.

I asked what course he'd done.
He explained the high-flying
Resolution of rootstock, the frailty
Of patrician grafts.

Next day he described
The enormous thirst of trees,
The flow of sap that makes each sprig
Stretch itself into leaves,
And how, in winter, each
Of these great drinkers shrinks
Inside its bark, thinks slow
Thoughts as the sun runs low.

Sandwich course? I suggested,
Job in municipal gardens?
A televisual career?
Why waste such talent here?

I haven't seen him since,
But I know where he's been;
Hollyhocks thoughtfully barbered
Before frost blacks their tops.

I know he's still around,
One day with kindest cuts
Dressing our shaggy borders;
Another, transplanted hydrangeas

Suddenly look at home.
Our scrubby grounds grow spruce.
Not much more left to do.
Will he start on the dwarfs next?

But he keeps clear of me.

ADMINISTRATOR

Underling too long, though finally you made it
To top dog, you knew the system too well
To bark authentically.

You, the expert on short cuts, on first-name terms
With the influential – stores, post-room, porters; you
Who knew how to fix it,

Whose good deeds were always shady, like
The fiddled day off for Christmas shopping, which
Was rightfully ours;

You who scrounged, never spent, who shook
With fright before committees, who always forgot
Your own authority;

Who dared not sanction our electric kettles,
Whose kindnesses were home-made, compensation
For your servile failure
To improve anything.

BACK TO THE FRONT

I remember too much here. Michaelmas daisies
Butterfly-bushed in September; ceanothus
That got above itself, the derelict caravan
Where I ate cheese and wrote on used paper.
A scorched-earth policy has scotched the lot.

Instead there are new toys, compact, intense,
User-unfriendly. The photocopier will mug me
If I face it alone. The phone is tapped
By a sharp inquisitor, who calculates my fear.
This wallpaper, with its lilt of country kitchens,
Was chosen to deceive.

O *you haven't changed!* say the ones who knew me
(Wanting not to have changed themselves).
But I have. I am older and more frightened.
Sophisticated engines run free in the kitchen,
Only the patients still huddle and fumble, and somewhere
Someone is still screaming.

And I ought to have been here yesterday,
They tell me, for six-foot Laura's language.
Words Averil had never heard before . . . We had to explain them.
The police had to come. *Yes*, they say, *yes,*
You would have enjoyed yesterday.

(Would I have ever enjoyed yesterday? Was I,
Before I went away, so good at relishing
The anger of the helpless, such an eaves-dropper
On misery? I suppose I was. I suppose that
Was how I lived, semi-attached to despair.)

And still unspoken misery slams through
Prim clinical diction. Doctors alone are still
The privileged, who *think* or *say;* patients
Are back at their old tricks, *claiming,*
Admitting, denying. Still they endure urinary urgency,
Demonstrate gait disturbance, suffer
Massive insults to the brain.

Saddest of all, the one who should remember;
The smart young man, always in and out of good jobs,
With his cavalier lovelocks, his way with women,
Slow, now, and spoiled. He doesn't like the shape
Of twenty-pence pieces. Can I change them for him?
I don't like the shape of your future, Tony.
No magician here can change the currency,
Or the fused charge in your head.

BUT, DOCTOR ...
A True Story about Confused Referral Letters

Sit down, my dear. I gather that you're not
Feeling too grand. So first things first. How are
Relations with your husband? Do you have
Orgasmic intercourse with him each night?
                              But Doctor, it's my feet . . .

Just move your chair a little more this way,
So that the telltale sun may show me all
The messages of lips, eyes, hands and skin,
The messages you dare not speak yourself.
                              But Doctor, it's my feet . . .

You are a woman. Do you feel fulfilled?
Do you go out to work, and so betray
Your feminine identity? Do you
Nurture your children? Are you on the Pill?
                              But Doctor, it's my feet . . .

Perhaps I shall prescribe another child,
Perhaps a fresher husband, or perhaps
(Your secret wish) I might prescribe a lover,
Extra-curricular, an understanding psy –
                              But Doctor, it's my feet . . .

Your tone, my child, is most significant.
Why so aggressive? And your fetishism
About your feet appears suspiciously
Deep-seated and deluded. Tell me all.
                              But Doctor, it's my feet . . .

Was masturbation early? And how far
Did your incestuous father push his love?
What makes you hate all men? When did you last
Murder your mother? Please be frank with me.
                    But Doctor, it's my feet . . .

Only together can we overcome
This dreadful trauma threatening to deprive
Your sovereignty of reason. Come, be brave.
. . . . Yes, Mrs Jones. You've got a nasty bunion.

CASEHISTORY: ALISON (HEAD INJURY)

(She looks at her photograph)

I would like to have known
My husband's wife, my mother's only daughter.
A bright girl she was.

Enmeshed in comforting
Fat, I wonder at her delicate angles.
Her autocratic knee

Like a Degas dancer's
Adjusts to the observer with airy poise,
That now lugs me upstairs

Hardly. Her face, broken
By nothing sharper than smiles, holds in its smiles
What I have forgotten.

She knows my father's dead,
And grieves for it, and smiles. She has digested
Mourning. Her smile shows it.

I, who need reminding
Every morning, shall never get over what
I do not remember.

Consistency matters.
I should like to keep faith with her lack of faith,
But forget her reasons.

Proud of this younger self,
I assert her achievements, her A levels,
Her job with a future.

Poor clever girl! I know,
For all my damaged brain, something she doesn't:
I am her future.

A bright girl she was.

CASEHISTORY: JULIE (ENCEPHALITIS)

She stands between us. Her dress
Is zipped up back to front.
She has been crying her eyes
Dark. Her legs are thinner than legs.

She is importunate.

I'm not mental, am I?
Someone told me I was mental,
But I lost me memory
'Cos our dad died.
It don't make sense though, do it?
After I've been a nurse.

Her speech is nothing.

If I been rude, I apologise.
I lost me memory
'Cos I had the flu, didn't I?
I thought it was 'cos our dad died, see.
But it was 'cos I had the flu.

What imports this song?

Married? O god forgive me.
Who to? Let's be fair,
If you're getting married,
You ought to know the man.
O, not Roy!
I didn't marry him, did I?
I must be mental.
I'll do meself in.

There is a willow.

He was different to my brothers.
God forgive me for saying this,
He was like a woman.
Children? O god, please help me,
Please do, god.

O rose of May.

I'm getting better,
The doctor told me so,
As god's me witness, touch wood.
O, I am hungry.
I hope you don't mind me asking,
Where's the toilet to?

Do you see this, O God?

What about me dad?
Me dad's not gone, is he?

CLERICAL ERROR

My raiment stinks of the poor and the afflicted,
Of those whom healers, in a parody of you,
Have called back to mimic life.

I understand they are yours, and concern
All of us. But I am paid to do other things.
What must I do when Job and his daughters

Cram into my office where they are not allowed,
When I am typing medical reports against the clock,
When they mop and mow at me, seeking comfort?

I can tell you what I do. I address them as *love*
(Which is an insult), and say in a special soothing voice
(Which fools no one), *Go to the nurses, Judith,*

Judith, the nurses are looking for you (which is a lie).
How, Sir, am I to reconcile this with your clear
Instructions on dealing with the afflicted

And the poor? I do not seek to justify
My job description. I did not write it,
But I volunteered to live by its commandments.

DEAR SIR

(in memory of Dr H. J. Crow)

Body prescribed a comic part for you,
Denied the pallor of those inchless, touchy men
Who terrorise worlds into taking them seriously,

Refused too the surgeon's histrionic profile,
Noble silver forelock, hairless fiddler's fingers.
Made you a shy Scot, haggis-shaped.

Laughter skirts the need for small-talk,
So you made yourself droll. Materialised
Tiptoeing round corners as Quack-in-the-box

(*Aha! Gotcher!*) short stout explosion
Cued to blast off in muffled thuds of laughter,
Your warning note down corridors a drone.

Gracefully at Christmas you accepted your vocation,
Assumed kilt, sporran, funny hat, the lot.
Little Lord Mis-Rule, whose considerate war-whoops

Shrouded your morbid clinical conscience.

But Sir, I accuse you of worrying about patients
After hours; of not sleeping; of irrational fears
For your children; of concealing your DFC courage;
Of inconspicuous valour on behalf of underdogs;
Of exploring humanity's dark places,
And not letting on; of making us all believe
We were curable; of mixing the genres,
Of playing Quixote in Sancho Panza's clothes.

And, Sir, I accuse you of losing heart,
Of not curing that endless queue of incurables,
Blight of Thursday afternoons; of believing they'd vanish
If you shut your eyes and wished.

O Sir, I accuse you of dying at home,
In bed, asleep, without a hint of impaired
Cortical integrity; of failing to present
An interesting case; of leaving no heir

To that florid prose style, to that susceptibility
To *Limehouse Blues* late on Fridays
In a subordinate's subtle hum.
                                        Dear Sir,
I accuse you of being irreplaceable. By God,
You had a crack at those windmills!

DICTATOR

He bestrides the wall-to-wall carpeting
Like a colossus. Imperiously
He surges from comma to semi-colon.

Swaying in the throes of his passionate
Dictation, he creates little draughts,
Which stir my piles of flimsy paper.

If my phone rings, he answers
In an assumed accent.

Flexing the muscles of his mind,
He rides in triumph through the agendas
Of Area and District Management Committees

Aborting all opposition with the flick
Of a fullstop. Laurelled and glossy
He paces the colonnades of an imperial future,
With all his enemies liquidated.

When his letters are typed, he forgets to sign them.

FOR SAINT PETER

I have a good deal of sympathy for you, mate,
Because I reckon that, like me, you deal with the outpatients.

Now the inpatients are easy, they're cowed by the nurses
(In your case, the angels) and they know what's what in the set-up.

They know about God (in my case Dr Snow) and all His little fads,
And if there's any trouble with them, you can easily scare them rigid

Just by mentioning His name. But outpatients are different.
They bring their kids with them, for one thing, and that creates a
    wrong atmosphere.

They have shopping baskets, and buses to catch. They cry, or knit,
Or fall on the floor in convulsions. In fact, Saint Peter,

If you know what I mean, they haven't yet learned
How to be reverent.

1974

FRIENDSHIP

Not soul-mates, exactly.
Their names say it all.

Chloe. Kylie. Normally
They wouldn't have met.
One poised, gentle, patient.
The other, a mum straight
From Nappy Valley. Both
Washed up on these sad shores,
Where the brain-damaged, the gibberers,
The obsessive, learn a difficult habit
Of living together,
                              but exclude
Scarred Chloe, who fell in the fire in a fit
And lost an eye, parts of her face;
Whose husband couldn't bear to see her.
And shaky Kylie, muttering endlessly
In the local patois, uncertain of everything:
Where was the canteen? When would her father
(Dead, of course) come to visit?
Hazy memories: who did I marry?
Children? All life's lovely things
Wiped clean by encephalitis. Husband, also,
Keeping clear.
                        What did they say,
One damaged thing to the other? Nobody
Wanted to ask, to talk to them.
But, as they drifted along corridors,
They were always chatting. Kylie feverishly,
Chloe listening with her old-fashioned courtesy,
Enlaced, arm-in-arm, like Victorian sisters,
Like friends.

FROM THE REMAND CENTRE

Eleven stone and nineteen years of want
Flex inside Koreen. Voices speak to her
In dreams of love. She needs it like a fag,
Ever since Mum, who didn't think her daft,
Died suddenly in front of her. She holds
Her warder lovingly with powerful palms,
Slings head upon her shoulders, cries *Get lost,*
Meaning *I love you*, and her blows caress.

IN MEMORY

The florist is sympathetic. She chooses
Chrysanthemums of a subfusc tone,
Contributes a card: *with deepest sympathy.*

The undertaker is sympathetic. He
Bares respectful teeth, folding our sad
Flowers close to his expensive black bosom.

The city is not sympathetic. It is
Abstracted. In grassed-over graveyards
Pigeons and children gobble potato crisps.

From vicarages and surgeries, wherever
Sensitive celibate men resort,
Come sensitive celibate sighs of relief.

For you are dead, who pursued them with tiepins,
Cufflinks, tasteful Medici postcards,
And quietly intense conversation. You are

Dead, passed away in your sleep in your chaste bed-
Sitter with the charming rural views.
Tomorrow you will be incinerated,

Like the October leaves. Only leaves return
In a secure succession, and you
Leave just a few embarrassing ashes.

You have much to forgive us. Will you try? We
Are the acquaintances you wanted
As friends, friends who avoided proper passion,

Lovers who preferred the cordiality
Of friendship. Your embers reproach us.
Forgive us our fear, who need professionals

To love and mourn for us, who spread our futile
Euphemisms over suicide,
And ask for pardon from the careless dead.

JOBDESCRIPTION: MEDICAL RECORDS

Innocence is important, and order.
You need have no truck with the
Seamy insides of notes, where blood
And malignant growths and indelicate

Photographs wait to alarm. We like
To preserve innocence. You will
Be safe here, under the permanent
Striplighting. (Twenty-four hours cover.

Someone is always here. Our notes
Require constant company.) No
Patients, of course. The porter comes
And goes, but doesn't belong. With

His hairless satyr's grin, he knows
More than is suitable. Your conversation
Should concern football and television.
You may laugh at his dirty jokes,

But not tell any. Operations
Are not discussed here. How, by
The way, is your imagination?
Poorly, I hope. We do not encourage

Speculation in clerks. We prefer you
To think of patients not as people, but
Digits. That makes it much easier. Our system
Is terminal digit filing. If you

Are the right type for us, you will be
Unconscious of overtones. The contrasting
Weights of histories (puffy
For the truly ill, thin and clean

For childhood's greenstick fractures)
Will not concern you. You will use
The Death Book as a matter of routine.
Our shelves are tall, our files heavy. Have you

A strong back and a good head for heights?

LAMENT FOR THE PATIENTS

These were far from lovely in their lives,
And when they died, they were instantly forgotten.

These were the permanent patients, the ones
Whose disease was living. Their trophy, death,
Being to no one's advantage, was kept dark.

These had quiet funerals (*no flowers,
Please*), silent incinerations, hushed-up autopsies;
Their dying figured in obituary columns
Of local papers only.

On these specialists had practised specialities;
Had weighed and measured; had taken samples
Of blood and urine; had tested IQs,
Reflexes, patience; had applied
Shock treatment, drugs and nice hot cups of tea.
Of these specialists had washed their hands,
Having failed to arrive at a satisfactory
Diagnosis (anglicè: having failed to infect them
With a reason for living). Therefore they died.

To me came the news of their dying:
From the police (*Was this individual
A patient of yours?*); from ambulance
Control (*Our team report this patient
You sent us to fetch is deceased already*);
From tight-lipped telephoning widowers
(*My wife died in her sleep last night*);
From carboned discharge letters (*I note
That you have preserved the brain. We would certainly
Be very interested in this specimen*);

From curt press cuttings (*Man found dead.*
Foul play not suspected). I annotated their notes
With their final symptom: *died.*
Therefore I remember them.

These I remember:
Sonia, David, Penny, who chose death.
Lynn and Gillian, who died undiagnosed.
Peter, whose death was enigmatic.
Simple Betty, who suddenly stopped living.
Lionhearted Gertrude, who persevered to the end.
Patricia, so sorry for herself,
For whom I was not sufficiently sorry.
Julian, the interesting case. Alan,
Broken by a lorry, resurrected by surgeons,
Who nevertheless contrived at length to die.

Not for these the proper ceremonies, the solemn crowds,
The stripped gun-carriage, the slow march from *Saul,*
The tumulus, the friendly possessions
At hand in the dark. Not even
The pauper's deal coffin, brief office
Of the uncared-for. Only the recital
Of disembodied voices in a clerk's ear,
A final emendation of the text.

LINGUIST

The smashed voice roars inside the ruined throat
Behind the mangled face. Voice of the wild,
Voice of the warthog calling to his mates,

Wordless, huge-volumed, sad. We can't make out
A meaning (though his wife can). Solitary
He sits, shrouded in his vast noise. How strange

To make so much, none of it any use
To fragile human ears, except to mis-
Inform. For we all make the obvious

And wrong deduction: *this poor chap is mad.*
He doesn't talk like us. He can't be sane.
And yet he is. Look in his serious eyes;

He understands. Reads magazines. He bawls
Obliterated meanings at his wife.
O yes, she says, *a sundial would be nice.*

That's what he'd like. A silent clock that speaks
The solemn language of the sun to grass
And garden-lovers with a turn for sums.

1974

MISS MORRIS

At seventy Miss Morris came to Death,
Who took her gently, as her time was up.
Her senile heart dealt with its final breath,
And then retired. But this old-fashioned cup
Was not allowed. Resourceful doctors tore
The dignity of dying from the dead;
Sinewy nurses flung her to the floor
And gave her cardiac massage. *Look*, they said,
There's something there. Defibrillation shocked
Her body, and she lived. She died again.
And lived. And died. And lived. Until she clocked
Her thirteenth resurrection, and in pain
Achieved extinction. Her life-saving bruises
Testify man can't die, until Man chooses.

1974

MODERN LAZARUS

(on the survivor of a car crash)

Triumphant doctors resurrected
This dead man.
Look, they said, no other age could
Do what this can.

He was dead. We have restored him
To moving life,
Returned him to his home and parents,
Children and wife.

This man's a monument to science.
We made him breathe.
We gave him back an eye. (The other
We had to leave.)

We gave him back his speech. (Well, almost.
It's true, it takes
Patience and skill to understand
The noise he makes.)

We couldn't give him back his brain
Brilliant and sure
But then, few people have minds such
As his, before.

Above all, we have recommended
Enormous sums
Be paid to him in compensation
And it's been done.

And so we claim that medicine
Which healed this man
Has never shown such godlike power
Since time began.

We thank you for your care and skill,
The quiet wife said
The cruel lorry was much kinder
It left him dead.

1974

NEUROLOGICAL INSTITUTE*

Her mother's flower arrangements humanise
The hospital. Outpatients like to see
Brush-headed teazels, beech leaves' blue disguise,
The round transparent heads of honesty.
No reek of ether here, no hint of blood;
Wall-to-wall carpets and two fat, spayed cats,
Somerset gardener, apple-trees in bud,
Healthy inpatients wearing woolly hats.

We operate on nothing trivial here;
We only amputate the anxious brain,
Excising cells until the knack of fear
Oozes away. That's why we're so urbane.
Our floral decor hints that you will find
Wall-to-wall carpeting within the mind.

1974

* also titled 'Woman's Touch'

NOT QUITE RIGHT

Excuse me, staff-lady, but I feel rotten hungry and
thirsty, honest, I feel really ill. I'm very sincerely
grateful for having my life saved. I'm not a fool.
I died once. My wife saved my life with the kiss of life.
I feel rotten hungry and thirsty. Would you have such a
thing on you as a piece of chewing-gum or a sweet?
Any chance of your lovely company for a game of crib?

Not the blunt planes of the dull-minded,
The junket façade of the deranged;
Sanity's fine dry-point composed this profile.
Above it, hemispheres in disorder.

O the higher up the mulberry tree
The sweeter grows the berry.

Not the doll's strut of the retarded,
The see-saw footing of the insane;
He runs our corridors lightly, like a boy,
Left arm bent, hand signalling a corner.
He is a motorbike. OOOO oooo

O the higher up the mulberry tree
The sweeter grows the cherry.

Not the candid eyeballs of imbeciles,
Lunacy's limp and slippery pupils;
Regal the gaze of his eye from its socket
As he angles his head to chat.

O the higher up the mulberry tree
The sweeter grows the parsley.

We swap jargon. I call him lad,
Naming him too often, like a dog.
He looks with his sane eyes. He speaks.
He says nothing.

O the higher up the mulberry tree
The sweeter grows the herring.

He shuffles his thoughts' thumbed pack.
No joker ever trumps the brain's dead cells.
Yet once when, bothered by his gibberish,
I said to him: *Say something cheerful, lad,*
For goodness' sake, he looked me in the eye
Wisely, and spoke: *I've got my life, I'm alive.*
I'm not a fool.

O the higher up the mulberry tree
The sweeter grows the berry.

OFF SICK

Regime of the house: the sun's morning
Tour, his unsuspected finger on a dim corner.

The house is not primed for my presence. I intrude
On its private life. Forgive me, house,

My excuse is fever. You can disregard me.
If I were myself I should not be here.

My true world is dancing to its own
Metronome: mail, first clinic, coffee-break,

FEM's letters. Someone there is being me,
Not perfectly, I hope. I sweat to think

They imagine me malingering, may fancy
I enjoy this fretting leisure, place of estrangement.

OLIVE

Generosity: the gift of the gods. This one
Is famous for giving Athens a singular tree.

We met in my office door. She'd jammed
Her hoover in it. *Sorry, my lover,* she said.

Don't like to leave it in the passage.
Patients fall over things. Daily thereafter

She'd hail me: *Still yur, then?* And once,
Thassa funny name you got. Latin, ennit? I'm Olive.

Now you know. Her first gift, drink. A cup of tea (hot)
By my phone every day when I came to work.

Thought you could do with it. All that way
Yew as to come. No kettle, ave yer?

Thought not. Not like they nurses,
Always at the Tetleys. Next came food

(A Welsh cake) on Fridays. *Nice recipe, ennit?*
Our Nan's. From the Forest, she wuz. After that, learning

(She was famous for it). *Bit ignorant about Bristol,*
Aren't yer? Ave a read of me book.

Later, understanding. *Yer won't learn much about patients*
From doctors and nurses. Yew as to get to like em.

We're in there ages doing them toilets. It all adds up.

She decided I needed laughter. Every day
Was waiting in my office with a joke,

Selected specially, just right for me –
Not rude or stale or obvious. Not easy, either.

She watched me like a suspect. Had I got there?
Or was my laugh just half a bar too late?

Her final gift was cryptic. She put
Three flaky bulbs in my hand when I left,

And *See what comes of they,* she said.
What came was lilies. Came, and keep on coming,

Tall and immortal in a mortal garden.

Note: Athene, the wise goddess, presented Athens with the
olive tree, the gift most useful to mortals.

ON A DEAD SOCIAL WORKER

She steered a firm course through equivocal
Currents, and spoke the language of the seas
Though her own dialect was different.
The shipwrecked liked her, hurled their sopping junk
On to her polished planks, and camped on board
Until they swamped the neat craft, and she foundered.

PATIENCE STRONG

Everyone knows her name. Trite calendars
Of rose-nooked cottages or winding ways
Display her sentiments in homespun verse
Disguised as prose. She has her tiny niche
In women's magazines, too, tucked away
Among the recipes or near the end
Of some perennial serial. Her theme
Always the same: rain falls in every life,
But rainbows, bluebirds, spring, babies or God
Lift up our hearts. No doubt such rubbish sells.
She must be feathering her inglenook.
Genuine poets seldom coin the stuff,
Nor do they flaunt such aptly bogus names.
Their message is oblique; it doesn't fit
A pocket diary's page; nor does it pay.

One day in epileptic outpatients,
A working-man, a fellow in his fifties,
Was feeling bad. I brought a cup of tea.
He talked about his family and job:
His dad was in the Ambulance Brigade;
He hoped to join, but being epileptic,
They wouldn't have him. *Naturally*, he said,
With my disease, I'd be a handicap.
But I'd have liked to help. He sucked his tea,
Then from some special inner pocket brought
A booklet muffled up in cellophane,
Unwrapped it gently, opened at a page –
Characteristic cottage garden, seen
Through chintzy casement windows. Underneath
Some cosy musing in the usual vein,
And *See*, he said, *this is what keeps me going.*

PATIENTS

Not the official ones, who have been
Diagnosed and made tidy. They are
The better sort of patient.

They know the answers to the difficult
Questions on the admission sheet
About religion, next of kin, sex.

They know the rules. The printed ones
In the *Guide for Patients*, about why we prefer
No smoking, the correct postal address;

Also the real ones, like the precise quota
Of servility each doctor expects,
When to have fits, and where to die.

These are not true patients. They know
Their way around, they present the right
Symptoms. But what can be done for us,

The undiagnosed? What drugs
Will help our Matron, whose cats are
Her old black husband and her young black son?

Who will prescribe for our nurses, fatally
Addicted to idleness and tea? What therapy
Will relieve our Psychiatrist of his lust

For young slim girls, who prudently
Pretend to his excitement, though age
Has freckled his hands and his breath smells old?

How to comfort our Director through his
Terminal distress, as he babbles of
Football and virility, trembling in sunlight?

There is no cure for us. O, if only
We could cherish our bizarre behaviour
With accurate clinical pity. But there are no

Notes to chart our journey, no one
Has even stamped CONFIDENTIAL or *Not to be
Taken out of the hospital* on our lives.

RESIGNATION LETTER

I am cartographer of the dull incline
Which all who visit choose to leave and forget.

I am on nodding terms with explorers of
The Rolandic Fissure, the Optic Chiasm, the Island of Reil.

I can guide the helpless to the lavatory,
The patients' canteen, the bus back to the centre.

I can interpret the hieroglyphs of initiates.
In the R 1/2 sphere the 9–10 Hz alpha rhythm

At 30–60 uv in amp. means nothing to me,
But I can decode it. My name is Pomp.

Circumstance is what I am paid to prevent.
It's all very well for you. Your sex life

Is probably all right is the sort of thing patients want
To shout at consultants. My job: to ensure that they don't.

I am keeper of keys and secrets. I am familiar
With high IQs and low grade mental defectives.

I am acquainted with the smells of grief,
Panic, obsession, incontinence, apathy.

I understand the meaning of expensive florists' bouquets
On patients' birthdays, and no visitors.

I know how to speak to ambulance men:
Flattery, gratitude, abject femininity. Never cap their jokes.

I have composed a full-scale commination service
For those who interrupt receptionists' coffee breaks,

Or say *Easy for some*. It is not easy.
I know too much, remember too much. It is time to go.

RESUSCITATION TEAM

Arrives like a jinn, instantly,
Equipped with beards, white coats, its own smell,
And armfuls of metal and rubber.

Deploys promptly round the quiet bed
With horseplay and howls of laughter.
We, who are used to life, are surprised

At this larky resurrection. Runs
Through its box of tricks, prick, poke and biff,
While we watch, amazed. The indifferent patient

Is not amused, but carries little weight,
Being stripped and fumbled
By so many rugger-players. My first corpse,

If she is a corpse, lies there showing
Too much breast and leg. The team
Rowdily throws up the sponge, demands soap and water,

Leaves at the double. One of us,
Uncertainly, rearranges the night-dress.
Is it professional to observe the proprieties

Now of her who leaves privately
Wheeled past closed doors, her face
Still in the rictus of victory?

SPRING AFTERNOON

The doves purr in the trees. The wild inmates
Of Stoke Park Mental Hospital next door
Shout their improper comments from barred windows.

Forsythia burns. Homely wallflowers breathe out
The smell of heaven. The nurses and the patients
Are taking tea in deckchairs in the garden,

Under the trees. Depressives and obsessives
Call gaily to us as they play at croquet.
The epileptics doze off in the grass.

Caged in normality, we dumbly watch
From our dark office windows, feel that something –
Spring? or our sanity? – has let us down.

SUPERANNUATED PSYCHIATRIST

Old scallywag scapegoat has skedaddled,
Retired at last to bridge and both kinds of bird-watching.
No more suspect phone calls from shady acquaintances,
Anonymous ladies and flush-faced Rotarians.

He could always be blamed when case-notes strayed.
(His MG boot? His mistress's bed? We enjoyed guessing.)
How we shall miss his reliable shiftiness,
Wow and flutter on tape, Wimbledon-fortnight illness,

Dr Macavity life. Dear foxy quack,
I relished your idleness, your improvisations,
Your faith in my powers of you-preservation.
Who will shoulder our errors now?

What of your replacement, the new high flyer,
Smelling of aftershave and ambition? Is that tic
Telling us something his mind will arrive at later?
Meantime, I watch his parentheses. A man so much given

To brackets is hedging his bets.

THE LIST

Flawlessly typed, and spaced
At the proper intervals,
Serene and lordly, they pace
Along tomorrow's list
Like giftbearers on a frieze.

In tranquil order, arrayed
With the basic human equipment –
A name, a time, a number –
They advance on the future.

Not more harmonious who pace
Holding a hawk, a fish, a jar
(The customary offerings)
Along the Valley of the Kings.

Tomorrow these names will turn nasty,
Senile, pregnant, late,
Handicapped, handcuffed, unhandy,
Muddled, moribund, mute,

Be stained by living. But here,
Orderly, equal, right,
On the edge of tomorrow, they pause
Like giftbearers on a frieze

With the proper offering,
A time, a number, a name.
I am the artist, the typist;
I did my best for them.

THE RECEPTIONIST

I'm the receptionist. I am an ear
That listens on the phone, a hand that makes
Appointments in the book, a pair of feet
To fetch you what you need. I am a room
Where you can pick and poke and use my phone,
My scissors and my paper. I am nothing.
I listen and I mark, but to no end.
Mistakes are mine, but nothing that's well done
By me is ever noticed. To be nothing
Has its own consolations. Mostly I am happy
But sometimes ear and hand and willing feet
And empty room know they are all one body
And intermesh. And I am Cerberus,
Guardian of Hell. Beware of me. I bite.

1974

THE RECEPTIONIST TO HER WATCH

Your job: to wake me with your tiny chime
(*De Camptown Racetrack*) at the proper time.
So what possessed you, that Outpatients day,
While I was holding a shaky hand, to come butting in with your
　　　　　endless, heartless *doo dah doo dah dey?*

THE WATCHER

I am a watcher; and the things I watch
Are birds and love.

Not the more common sorts of either kind.
Not sparrows, nor

Young couples. Such successful breeds are blessed
By church and state,

Surviving in huge quantities. I like
The rare Welsh kite,

Clinging to life in the far Radnor hills;
The tiny wren,

Too small for winter; and the nightingale,
Chased from her home

By bulldozers and speculating men.
In human terms,

The love I watch is rare, its habitat
Concealed and strange.

The very old, the mad, the failures. These
Have secret shares

Of loving and of being loved. I can't
Lure them with food,

Stare at them through binoculars, or join
Societies

That will preserve them. Birds are easier
To do things for.

But love is so persistent, it survives
With no one's help.

Like starlings in Trafalgar Square, cut off
By many miles

From life-supporting trees, finding their homes
On dirty roofs,

So these quiet lovers, miles from wedding bells,
Cherish their odd

And beastly dears with furtive fondling hands
And shamefaced looks,

Finding their nesting-place in hospitals
And prison cells.

TRANSITIONAL OBJECT

Sits, holding nurse's hard reassuring hand
In her own two small ones.

Is terrified. Mews in her supersonic
Panic voice: *Help. Help. Please.*

Cries for Mummy, Daddy, Philip, the bus. Tries
To get up, to escape.

Is restrained by adult, would-be comforting
Hands and arms. Fights them.

Is brought a sweet warm drink, and is too shaky
With fear to swallow it.

The nurse cuddles her, snuggles the young amber
Ringlets against the grey.

Is not to be consoled. Her only comfort
The white blanket she hugs.

Whispers, *Help. Help. Please.* Cries for Mummy, Daddy,
Philip. She is 83,

Resisting childhood as it closes in.

TYPIST

She sitteth among the cymbals.
She clasheth the loud cymbals.

Men's faded voices twitter
Their dreams in her brusque ears.
Automatically she corrects their grammar.

Her drawer holds bright sharp things
That cut, punch, prick, impale.
She has a deadly way with a knife.
She can kill paper.

She sitteth among the cymbals.

Mistress of words,
She summons voices from the world's end
With one finger.

Benighted in the glacier of their scorn,
Her masters' jolly grins
Freeze their cheekbones.

She clasheth the loud cymbals.

One day she will speak her mind
In perfect grammar. One day she will snip
Their tapes with her scissor.

One day she will rise with all her sisters
Their war cry will be QWERTYUIOP.
They will kill men.

She sitteth among the cymbals.
She clasheth the loud cymbals.

WAITING

The porter blows his nose with two fingers
In a clinical way.

The nurses giggle when they meet. They have permission to do this.
That is how we know they are nurses.

The receptionist addresses the telephone by its Christian name.
She too is part of the inner circle.

There are two consultants. Occasionally they walk the room.
They are never able to speak.

A great many bit-part players, the outpatients
Have come unprepared. No one has told them
That this is a serious play, they have major parts.
They chat about floods in the Severn valley, softly they practise
breathing.

The worst of all, the man on the stretcher, the woman who
cannot walk,
Are the most at ease. They are the ones
Whom the nurses already know. Who smile, and tease,
Knowing they have reached the last act.